Journey to Healing

And the **POWER** of the **LORD** was present to **HEAL** them.
Luke 5:17

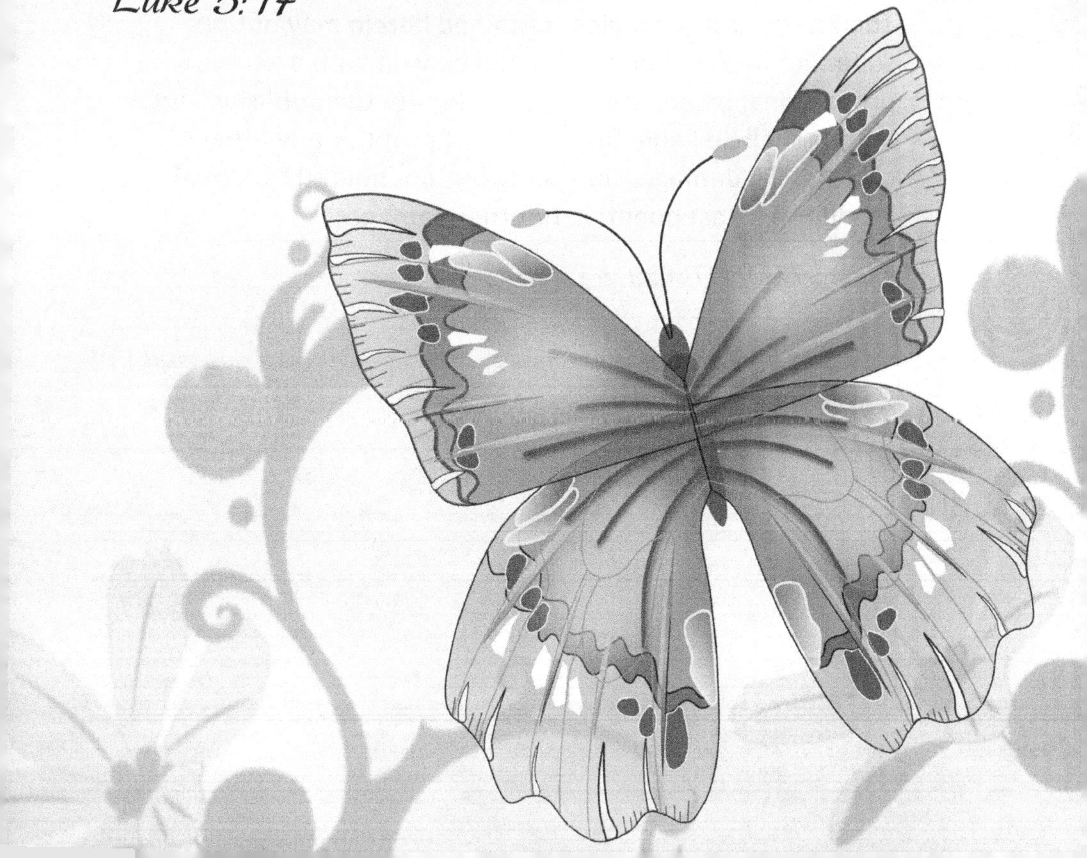

ISBN: 978-0-9976639-2-1

HOW TO USE THIS BOOK:

First, I know this is not easy and my prayers are with you. Although this is not something any woman wants to endure, nevertheless, you have come to a point in time where your healing and recovery is a priority.

This journal starts with your consultation with your physician so you'll have an accurate record of the procedure(s) that you will undergo. I start here because as you go through your recovery(your care and treatment), it will not be like anyone else's and it's always important to understand the next step that will be required.

Journaling has also been known to be therapeutic.

Date of Visit: ____________________

Doctor's Name: ____________________

← Date & Doctor Information

Notes:

____
____
____
____
____
____
____
____
____
____
____
____
____

← Jot down pertinent notes during your doctor visit.

HOW TO USE THIS BOOK cont'd:

I share an encouraging scripture or quote for the day.

The *Express Section* is an area to journal your emotions throughout your day. After you write down your emotions, please meditate and pray about whatever's concerning you at this time.

Scripture/Quote:

Encouraging Scripture or Quote for the day.

[Thoughts, Meditation & Prayer]

Jot down exactly the emotions you're experiencing.

Spend some quiet time meditating and praying about what you're experiencing.

Date of Visit: ___________________________

Doctor's Name: ___________________________

Notes:

Scripture/Quote for the day

"O Lord, if you heal me, I will be truly healed; if you save me, I will be truly saved. My praises are for you alone!" ~Jeremiah 17:14

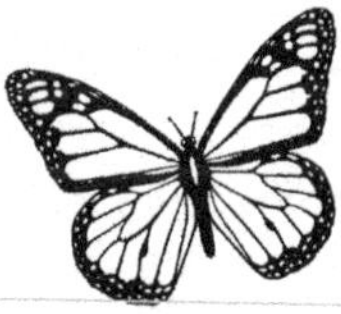

[Thoughts, Meditation & Prayer]

Date of Visit: ______________________________

Doctor's Name: ______________________________

Notes:

Scripture/Quote for the day

"Prayer is not asking. Prayer is putting oneself in the hands of God, at His disposition, and listening to His voice in the depth of our hearts." ~Mother Teresa

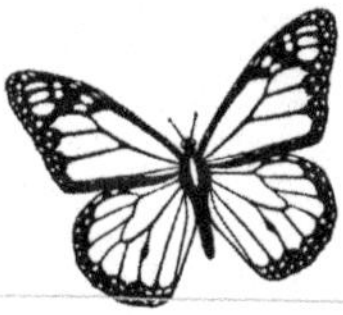

[Thoughts, Meditation & Prayer]

Date of Visit: ______________________________

Doctor's Name: ____________________________

Notes:

<u>Scripture/Quote for the day</u>

"Don't be afraid, for I am with you. Don't be discouraged, for I am your God. I will strengthen you and help you; I will hold you up with my victorious right hand." ~Isaiah 41:10

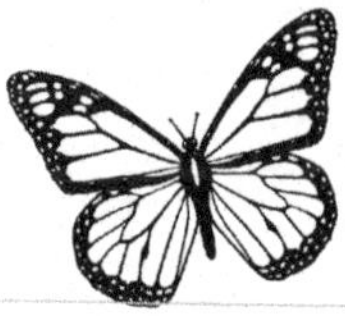

[Thoughts, Meditation & Prayer]

Date of Visit: ____

Doctor's Name: ____

Notes:

Scripture/Quote for the day

"Faith does not eliminate questions. But faith knows where to take them." ~Elisabeth Elliot

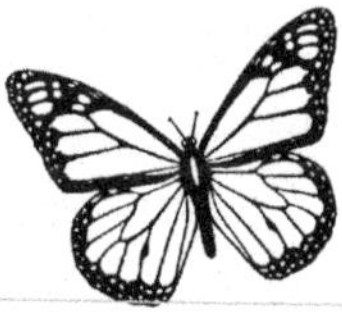

[Thoughts, Meditation & Prayer]

Date of Visit: ____

Doctor's Name: ____

Notes:

Scripture/Quote for the day

Then Jesus said, "Come to me, all you who are weary and carry heavy burdens, and I will give you rest." ~Matthew 11:28

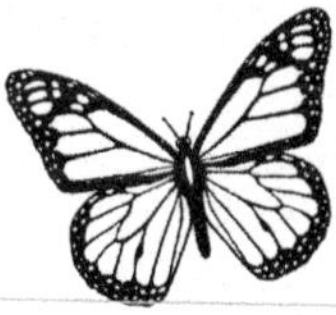

[Thoughts, Meditation & Prayer]

Date of Visit: ______________________________________

Doctor's Name: ____________________________________

Notes:

Scripture/Quote for the day

"You're stronger than you know, braver than you think, more loved than you can imagine." ~Roz

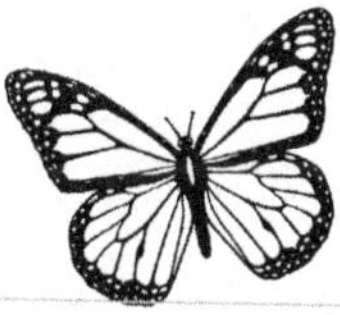

[Thoughts, Meditation & Prayer]

Date of Visit: ___________________________________

Doctor's Name: _________________________________

Notes:

Scripture/Quote for the day

"He heals the brokenhearted and bandages their wounds."

~Psalm 147:3

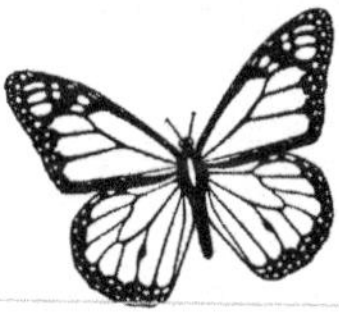

[Thoughts, Meditation & Prayer]

Date of Visit: ___________________________

Doctor's Name: ___________________________

Notes:

Scripture/Quote for the day

"What gives me the most hope every day is God's grace; knowing that his grace is going to give me the strength for whatever I face, knowing that nothing is a surprise to God." ~Rick Warren

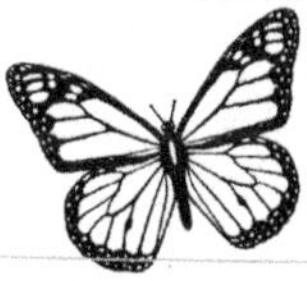

[Thoughts, Meditation & Prayer]

Date of Visit: ______________________________

Doctor's Name: ______________________________

Notes:

Scripture/Quote for the day

"The Sovereign Lord is my strength! He makes me as surefooted as a deer, able to tread upon the heights." ~*Habakkuk 3:19*

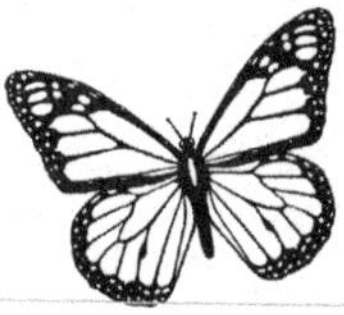

[Thoughts, Meditation & Prayer]

Date of Visit: ______________________________

Doctor's Name: ______________________________

Notes:

Scripture/Quote for the day

"No matter what you look like or think you look like you're special and loved and perfect just the way you are." ~Ariel Winter

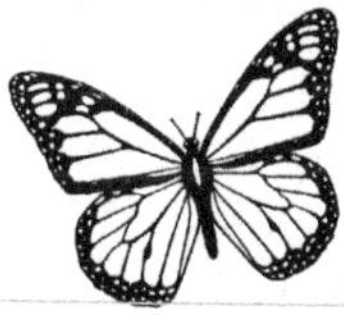

[Thoughts, Meditation & Prayer]

Date of Visit: ___________________________

Doctor's Name: ___________________________

Notes:

Scripture/Quote for the day

"Pleasant words are like a honeycomb, Sweetness to the soul and health to the bones." ~Proverbs 16:24

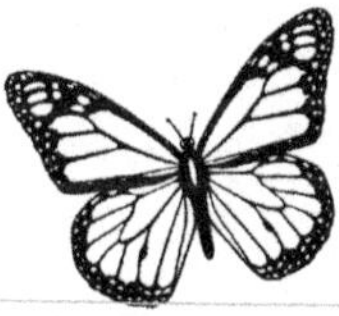

[Thoughts, Meditation & Prayer]

Date of Visit: ______________________________

Doctor's Name: ______________________________

Notes:

Scripture/Quote for the day

"What lies behind us and what lies before us are small matters compared to what lies within us." ~Ralph Waldo Emerson

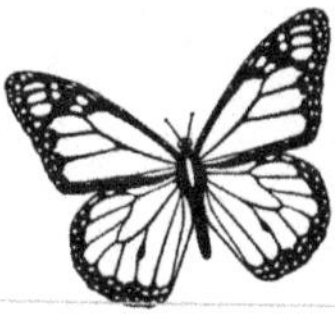

[Thoughts, Meditation & Prayer]

Date of Visit: ___________________________

Doctor's Name: ___________________________

Notes:

Scripture/Quote for the day

"Dear friend, I hope all is well with you and that you are as healthy in body as you are strong in spirit." ~3 John 1:2

[Thoughts, Meditation & Prayer]

Date of Visit: ______________________________

Doctor's Name: ______________________________

Notes:

Scripture/Quote for the day

"A happy person is not a person in a certain set of circumstances, but rather a person with a certain set of attitudes." ~Hugh Downs

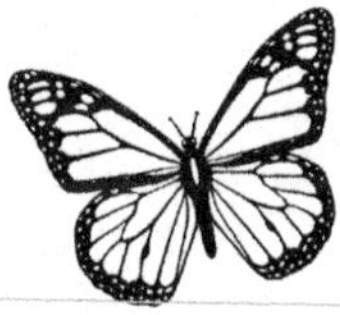

[Thoughts, Meditation & Prayer]

Date of Visit: ______________________________

Doctor's Name: ______________________________

Notes:

<u>Scripture/Quote for the day</u>

"O LORD my God, I cried to you for help and you restored my health." ~Psalm 30:2

[Thoughts, Meditation & Prayer]

Date of Visit: ____________________

Doctor's Name: ____________________

Notes:

Scripture/Quote for the day

"My home is in Heaven. I'm just traveling through this world."

~Billy Graham

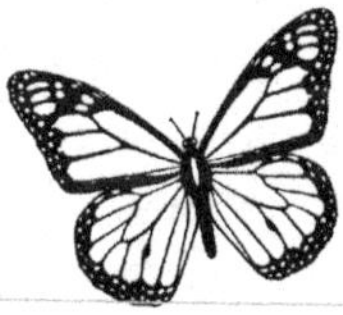

[Thoughts, Meditation & Prayer]

Date of Visit: ___________________________

Doctor's Name: ___________________________

Notes:

Scripture/Quote for the day

"And my God shall supply all your need according to His riches in glory by Christ Jesus." ~*Philippians 4:19*

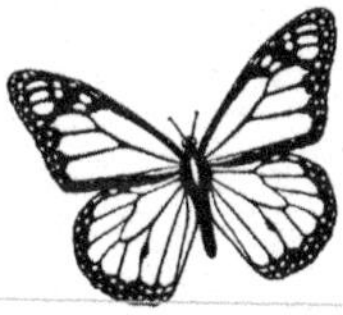

[Thoughts, Meditation & Prayer]

Date of Visit: ____

Doctor's Name: ____

Notes:

Scripture/Quote for the day

"Worry does not empty tomorrow of its sorrow. It empties today of its strength." ~Corrie ten Boom

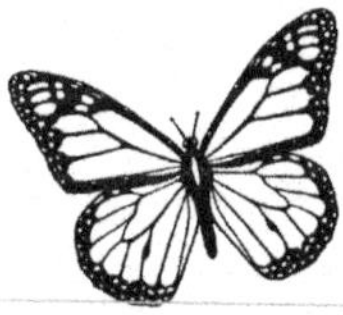

[Thoughts, Meditation & Prayer]

Date of Visit: ______________________________

Doctor's Name: ______________________________

Notes:

Scripture/Quote for the day

"Behold, I will bring to it health and healing, and I will heal them and reveal to them abundance of peace and truth." ~*Jeremiah 33:6*

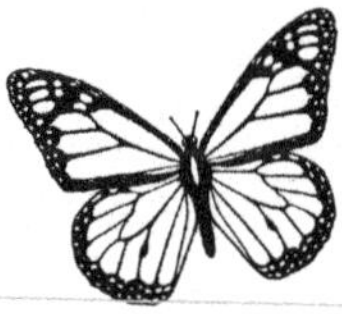

[Thoughts, Meditation & Prayer]

Date of Visit: ___

Doctor's Name: ___

Notes:

Scripture/Quote for the day

"The greatest act of faith some days is to simply get up and face another day." ~Amy Gatliff

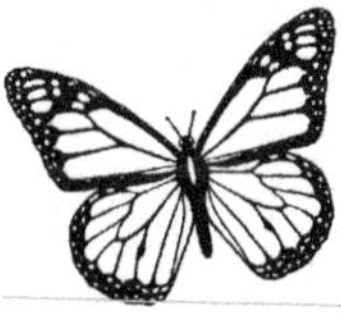

[Thoughts, Meditation & Prayer]

Date of Visit: ______________________________

Doctor's Name: ______________________________

Notes:

Scripture/Quote for the day

"Yet it was our weaknesses he carried; it was our sorrows that weighed him down. And we thought his troubles were a punishment from God, a punishment for his own sins! But he was pierced for our rebellion, crushed for our sins. He was beaten so we could be whole. He was whipped so we could be healed." ~Isaiah 53:4-5

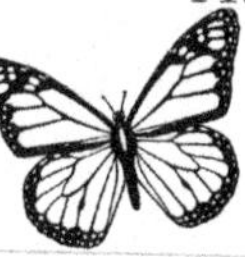

[Thoughts, Meditation & Prayer]

Date of Visit: ______________________________

Doctor's Name: ______________________________

Notes:

Scripture/Quote for the day

"Life is not measured by the number of breaths we take, but by the ***moments that take our breath away.****"* *~Maya Angelou*

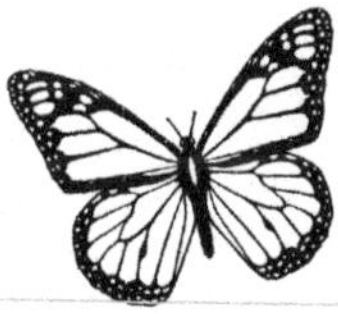

[Thoughts, Meditation & Prayer]

Date of Visit: ______________________________

Doctor's Name: ______________________________

Notes:

Scripture/Quote for the day

"This is my command—be strong and courageous! Do not be afraid or discouraged. For the Lord your God is with you wherever you go." ~*Joshua 1:9*

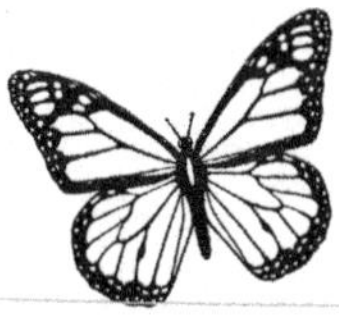

[Thoughts, Meditation & Prayer]

Date of Visit: ____________________________________

Doctor's Name: __________________________________

Notes:

Scripture/Quote for the day

"The most common way people give up their power is ***by thinking they don't have any."*** *~Alice Walker*

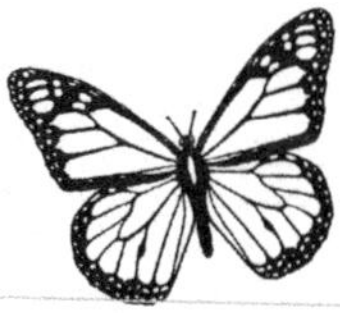

[Thoughts, Meditation & Prayer]

Date of Visit: ______________________________

Doctor's Name: ______________________________

Notes:

Scripture/Quote for the day

"So be strong and courageous all you who put your hope in the Lord." ~Psalm 31:24

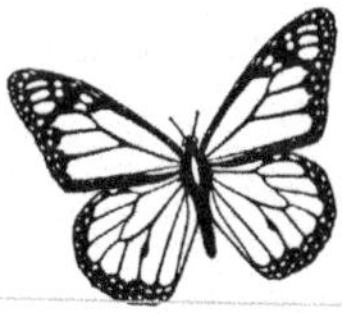

[Thoughts, Meditation & Prayer]

Date of Visit: ___________________________

Doctor's Name: ___________________________

Notes:

Patient Name

Doctor's Name

N

Scripture/Quote for the day

*"The best and **most beautiful things in the world cannot be seen nor touched** but are felt in the heart."* ~Helen Keller

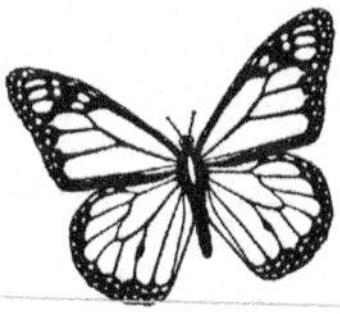

[Thoughts, Meditation & Prayer]

Date of Visit: ______________________________

Doctor's Name: ______________________________

Notes:

Scripture/Quote for the day

"And the POWER of the LORD was present to HEAL them"

~Luke 5:17

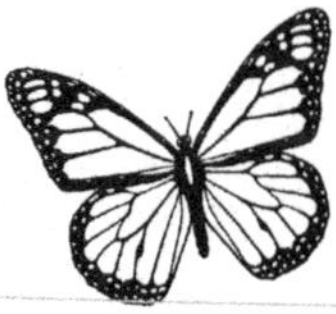

[Thoughts, Meditation & Prayer]

Date of Visit: ______________________________

Doctor's Name: ______________________________

Notes:

Scripture/Quote for the day

"Let God's promises shine on your problems." ~Corrie ten Boom

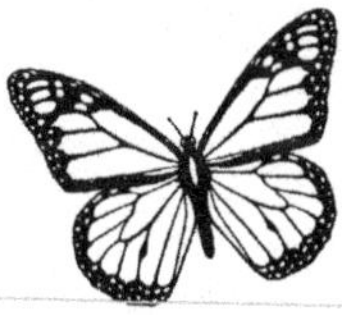

[Thoughts, Meditation & Prayer]

Date of Visit: ____

Doctor's Name: ____

Notes:

Scripture/Quote for the day

"I know the Lord is always with me. I will not be shaken, for he is right beside me." ~*Psalm 16:8*

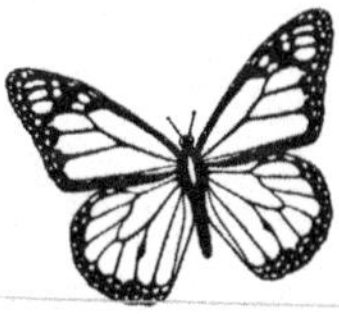

[Thoughts, Meditation & Prayer]

Date of Visit: ______________________________

Doctor's Name: ______________________________

Notes:

Scripture/Quote for the day

"Relying on God has to start all over everyday, as if nothing has yet been done." ~C. S. Lewis

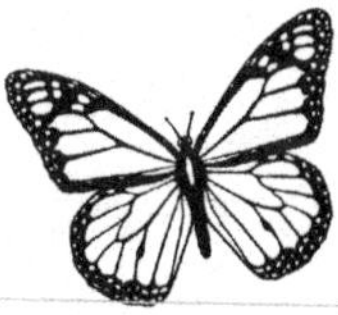

[Thoughts, Meditation & Prayer]

Date of Visit: ______________________________

Doctor's Name: ______________________________

Notes:

Scripture/Quote for the day

"Give all your worries and cares to God, for he cares about you."

~1 Peter 5:7

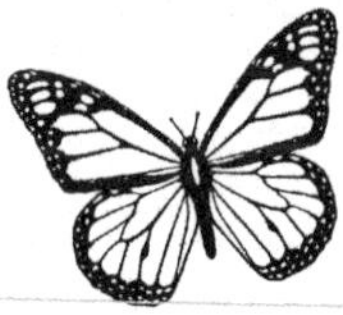

[Thoughts, Meditation & Prayer]

Date of Visit: ___________________________________

Doctor's Name: ___________________________________

Notes:

Scripture/Quote for the day

"There is no one who is insignificant in the purpose of God."

~Alistair Begg

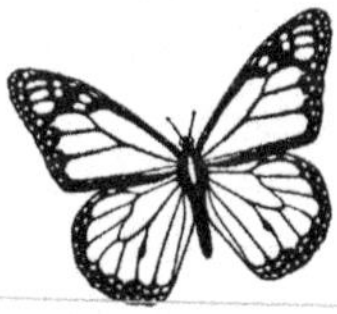

[Thoughts, Meditation & Prayer]

Date of Visit: ________________________________

Doctor's Name: ______________________________

Notes:

Scripture/Quote for the day

"You will keep in perfect peace all who trust in you, all whose thoughts are fixed on you!" ~Isaiah 26:3

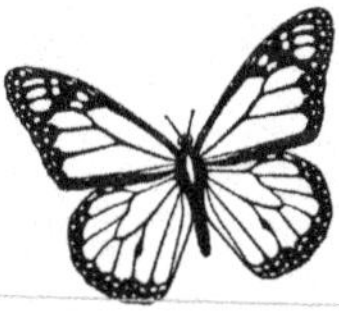

[Thoughts, Meditation & Prayer]

Date of Visit: ______________________________

Doctor's Name: ______________________________

Notes:

Scripture/Quote for the day

"HIS is a loving, tender hand, full of sympathy and compassion."

~D.L. Moody

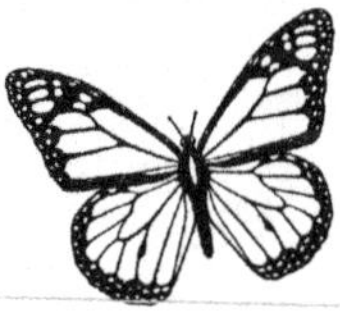

[Thoughts, Meditation & Prayer]

Date of Visit: ______________________________

Doctor's Name: ______________________________

Notes:

Scripture/Quote for the day

"In my distress I cried to the Lord, And He heard me." ~Psalm 120:1

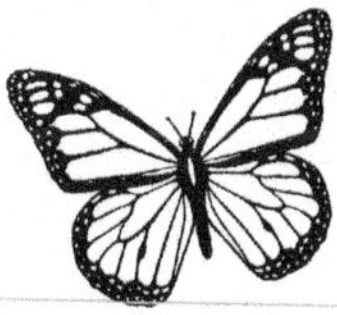

[Thoughts, Meditation & Prayer]

Date of Visit: ______________________________

Doctor's Name: ______________________________

Notes:

Scripture/Quote for the day

"The best use of life is love. The best expression of love is time. The best time to love is now." ~Rick Warren

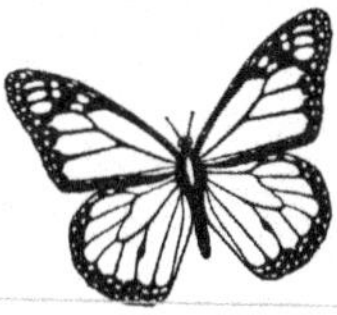

[Thoughts, Meditation & Prayer]

Date of Visit: ___________________________________

Doctor's Name: ________________________________

Notes:

Scripture/Quote for the day

"Give your burdens to the Lord, and He will take care of you. He will not permit the godly to slip and fall." ~*Psalm 55:22*

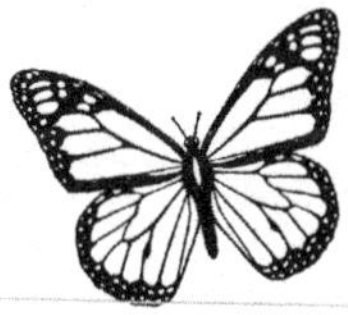

[Thoughts, Meditation & Prayer]

Date of Visit: ______________________________

Doctor's Name: ______________________________

Notes:

Scripture/Quote for the day

"Laughter is the most beautiful and beneficial therapy God ever granted humanity." ~Chuck Swindoll

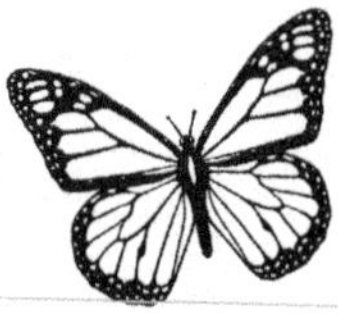

[Thoughts, Meditation & Prayer]

Date of Visit: ______________________________

Doctor's Name: ______________________________

Notes:

Scripture/Quote for the day

"I have told you all this so that you may have peace in me. Here on earth you will have many trials and sorrows. But take heart, because I have overcome the world." ~John 16:33

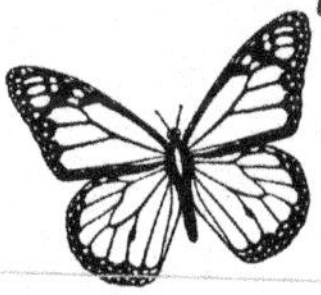

[Thoughts, Meditation & Prayer]

Date of Visit: ____________________

Doctor's Name: ____________________

Notes:

Scripture/Quote for the day

"It is impossible for that man to despair who remembers that his Helper is omnipotent." ~Jeremy Taylor

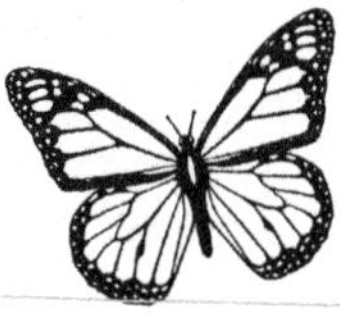

[Thoughts, Meditation & Prayer]

Date of Visit: ______________________________

Doctor's Name: ______________________________

Notes:

Scripture/Quote for the day

"I am leaving you with a gift–peace of mind and heart. And the peace I give is a gift the world cannot give. So don't be troubled or afraid." ~John 14:27

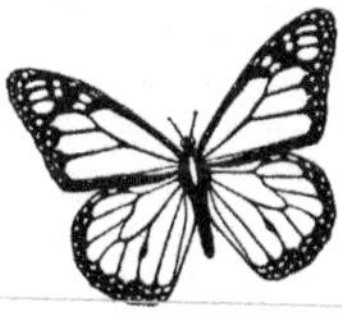

[Thoughts, Meditation & Prayer]

Date of Visit: ____

Doctor's Name: ____

Notes:

Scripture/Quote for the day

"God is most glorified in us when we are most satisfied in Him."
~John Piper

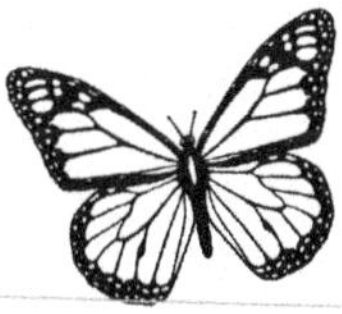

[Thoughts, Meditation & Prayer]

Date of Visit: ______________________________

Doctor's Name: ______________________________

Notes:

Scripture/Quote for the day

"The name of the LORD is a strong fortress; the godly run to him and are safe." ~*Proverbs 18:10*

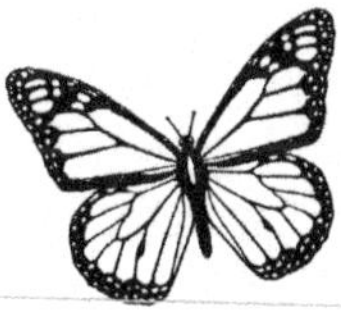

[Thoughts, Meditation & Prayer]

Date of Visit: ______________________________

Doctor's Name: ______________________________

Notes:

Scripture/Quote for the day

"Prayer is the link that connects us with God." ~A.B. Simpson

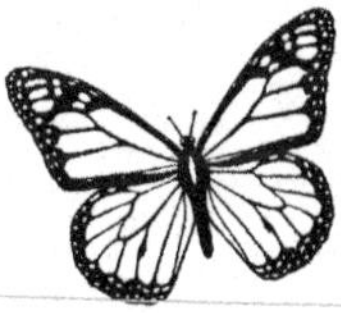

[Thoughts, Meditation & Prayer]

Date of Visit: ____________________

Doctor's Name: ____________________

Notes:

Scripture/Quote for the day

"I can do all things through Christ who strengthens me."

~Philippians 4:13

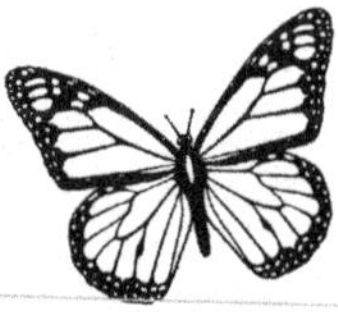

[Thoughts, Meditation & Prayer]

Date of Visit: ______________________________

Doctor's Name: ______________________________

Notes:

Scripture/Quote for the day

"Prayer is simply a two-way conversation between you and God."

~Billy Graham

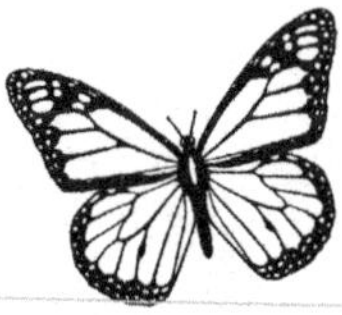

[Thoughts, Meditation & Prayer]

Dedication

You are a beautiful, phenomenal woman of God, precious to Him in every way. As you continue on your healing journey, know that He will increase your strength by allowing you to lean on His never-ending affection. His presence can cast out any weakness and guide you through every circumstance and decision you face, if you allow Him.

Use this journal to record that journey, to express your thoughts, to meditate and pour out your prayers, and in turn hear God's whispers of love and support.

Be strong in the Lord and may His unfailing love guide your heart into a fearless future.

Your friend,

Roz

RozBennerman.com

Made in the USA
Monee, IL
04 November 2026

67383420R00105